CIALIS

The Untold Story Of A Breakthrough ED
Medication, Exploring Its Origins,
Pharmacological Marvels, And Pioneering
Role In Redefining Male Potency,
Romance, And Beyond

Dr. Young Robinson

Contents

CHAPTER 1

INTRODUCTION TO ERECTILE DYSFUNCTION AND TREATMENT OPTIONS

Erectile dysfunction (ED) is a common condition that affects millions of men worldwide. It refers to the persistent inability to achieve or maintain an erection sufficient for satisfactory sexual performance. While ED can have physical, psychological, or lifestyle-related causes, its impact on self-esteem, relationships, and overall quality of life is profound.

In recent decades, the medical community has made significant strides in developing effective treatments for ED. This chapter serves as an introduction to the world of ED and provides an overview of the various treatment options available.

UNDERSTANDING THE PREVALENCE AND IMPACT OF ERECTILE DYSFUNCTION

ED is more prevalent than commonly thought, affecting men of all ages. While it becomes more common as men age, it is not exclusive to older individuals. Lifestyle factors such as stress, obesity, smoking, and lack of exercise can contribute to the development of ED. Additionally, medical conditions like diabetes, hypertension, and cardiovascular disease are known to increase the risk of ED.

EXPLORING DIFFERENT TREATMENT APPROACHES

Traditionally, ED treatments included psychotherapy, vacuum constriction devices, and intracavernosal injections. However, the advent of oral medications marked a turning point in ED treatment. The introduction of PDE5 inhibitors revolutionized the landscape by providing a more convenient and effective solution for many men.

INTRODUCING CIALIS AS A POPULAR ED MEDICATION

One of the most notable PDE5 inhibitors is Cialis, generically known as tadalafil. Cialis gained popularity due to its unique duration of action, often referred to as the "weekend pill." Unlike other PDE5 inhibitors, Cialis can provide effects lasting up to 36 hours, allowing for greater spontaneity in sexual activities.

THE SCIENCE BEHIND CIALIS: MECHANISM OF ACTION

To comprehend the effectiveness of Cialis in treating erectile dysfunction, it's essential to understand its mechanism of action. At the core of Cialis's function lies the enzyme phosphodiesterase type 5 (PDE5), which plays a pivotal role in regulating blood flow to the penis.

PDE5 AND ITS ROLE IN ERECTILE DYSFUNCTION

PDE5 is an enzyme that breaks down cyclic guanosine monophosphate (cGMP), a molecule responsible for relaxing the smooth muscle cells within blood vessel walls. In individuals with ED, the production of cGMP is compromised, leading to inadequate relaxation of these muscle cells. This constriction of blood vessels results in reduced blood flow to the penis, making it difficult to achieve and maintain an erection.

CIALIS'S SELECTIVE INHIBITION OF PDE5

Cialis, or tadalafil, is a PDE5 inhibitor. It works by blocking the action of PDE5, allowing cGMP levels to accumulate. As a result, the smooth muscle cells relax, blood vessels dilate, and blood flow to the penis increases. This enhanced blood flow enables the penile tissue to engorge with blood, resulting in a firm and lasting erection.

UNIQUE FEATURES OF CIALIS'S MECHANISM

What sets Cialis apart from other PDE5 inhibitors is its extended duration of action. While other medications in this class typically provide effects for 4 to 6 hours, Cialis can offer its benefits for up to 36 hours. This characteristic has earned Cialis the nickname "the weekend pill," as it allows couples greater flexibility in timing their sexual activities.

BENEFITS AND LIMITATIONS OF CIALIS

Cialis, with its unique characteristics and mechanism of action, offers several benefits as well as certain limitations that individuals should be aware of before use. In this chapter, we'll delve into these aspects to help you make an informed decision about incorporating Cialis into your treatment plan for erectile dysfunction.

ADVANTAGES OF CIALIS

1. **Extended Duration:** As previously mentioned, one of the standout features of Cialis is its prolonged effectiveness,

lasting up to 36 hours. This extended window provides more flexibility for intimate moments, allowing couples to engage in sexual activities without strict time constraints.

2. **Spontaneity:** Due to its longer duration of action, users can take Cialis well before the anticipated sexual activity, reducing the need to plan for the medication's timing.

3. **Daily Use Option:** In addition to the as-needed formulation, Cialis is available in a daily dose for those who prefer regular dosing. This option can provide continuous improvement in erectile function, potentially eliminating the need to time medication use.

CHAPTER 2

LIMITATIONS AND CONSIDERATIONS

1. **Delayed Onset:** While Cialis offers a longer duration of action, it may take longer to take effect compared to other PDE5 inhibitors. Users should be aware of this delayed onset and plan accordingly.

2. **Potential Side Effects:** Like any medication, Cialis can cause side effects. Common side effects include headache, indigestion, muscle aches, and nasal congestion. Severe side effects are rare but possible.

3. **Not Suitable for Everyone:** Cialis may not be suitable for individuals with certain medical conditions or those

taking specific medications. It's crucial to consult a healthcare professional before starting Cialis to ensure it is safe and appropriate.

4. **Cost:** The cost of Cialis can vary, and insurance coverage may vary as well. Considering the financial aspect is important when choosing an ED treatment.

DOSAGE, ADMINISTRATION, AND TIMING OF CIALIS

Choosing the right dosage, understanding how to administer Cialis, and timing its usage correctly are essential factors in maximizing the medication's effectiveness while minimizing potential risks. In this chapter, we'll delve into these important aspects.

SELECTING THE RIGHT DOSAGE

Cialis is available in various dosages, typically ranging from 2.5 mg to 20 mg. The appropriate dosage depends on factors such as the severity of your erectile dysfunction, your overall health, and your response to the medication. Starting with a lower dose and adjusting it as needed is a common approach to find the optimal balance between effectiveness and side effects.

ADMINISTRATION METHODS

Cialis comes in two primary formulations: the as-needed version and the daily use version.

1. **As-Needed Cialis:** This formulation is taken shortly before anticipated sexual activity. The effects can last for up to 36 hours, offering flexibility in timing. It's

important to note that sexual stimulation is still necessary for the medication to work. The recommended starting dose is often 10 mg.

2. **Daily Cialis:** This version involves taking a lower dose of Cialis every day, regardless of sexual activity. This can lead to more consistent improvements in erectile function over time. The daily dose is typically lower, such as 2.5 mg or 5 mg.

TIMING CONSIDERATIONS

For as-needed Cialis, timing is crucial. Taking the medication about 30 minutes to an hour before sexual activity is generally recommended. This allows sufficient time for the medication to take effect. Keep in mind that individual response times can vary, so experimenting with timing may be necessary.

Daily Cialis, on the other hand, doesn't require precise timing around sexual activity. Since it's taken regularly, it helps maintain a baseline level of the medication in your system, potentially providing more consistent erectile function improvement.

As we move forward, we'll share real-life success stories and patient experiences, helping you gain

REAL-LIFE SUCCESS STORIES AND PATIENT EXPERIENCES WITH CIALIS

Real stories from individuals who have experienced the positive impact of Cialis can provide valuable insights and inspiration for those considering the medication as a treatment option for erectile dysfunction. In this chapter, we'll share a variety of personal experiences to showcase the emotional and practical aspects of using Cialis.

PERSONAL ANECDOTES OF IMPROVEMENT

Individuals who have successfully incorporated Cialis into their lives often report significant improvements in their sexual experiences. They highlight the restoration of confidence, intimacy, and spontaneity that they had lost due to erectile dysfunction. By sharing these stories, readers can understand the emotional transformation that can occur when ED is effectively treated.

COUPLES' PERSPECTIVES

Success stories are not only about the individuals using Cialis but also about the impact on their partners. Partners often express how the improved sexual health has positively affected their relationships, leading to enhanced communication, emotional connection, and overall satisfaction.

CHAPTER 3

ADDRESSING EMOTIONAL WELL-BEING

Beyond the physical benefits, Cialis can also contribute to the emotional well-being of individuals and couples. Overcoming the challenges of erectile dysfunction can alleviate stress, anxiety, and feelings of inadequacy, resulting in a more positive outlook on life and relationships.

BALANCING EXPECTATIONS

While success stories are inspiring, it's important to remember that individual experiences can vary. Not everyone will have the same results, and there might be instances where Cialis might not work as desired. Realistic expectations, open communication with healthcare providers, and an understanding of the potential limitations of the medication are essential.

CIALIS AND BEYOND: FUTURE TRENDS AND RESEARCH

As science and medicine continue to advance, the field of erectile dysfunction treatment is not exempt from innovation and ongoing research. This chapter delves into the exciting developments, emerging trends, and potential breakthroughs that could shape the future of ED treatment, including the role of Cialis.

EXPLORING ADVANCEMENTS IN ED TREATMENT

The treatment landscape for erectile dysfunction has evolved significantly over the past few decades, with PDE5 inhibitors like Cialis representing a major leap forward.

However, the journey doesn't end here. Ongoing research aims to refine existing treatments and explore novel approaches to addressing ED.

GENE THERAPY AND REGENERATIVE MEDICINE

One promising avenue of research involves gene therapy and regenerative medicine. Scientists are investigating ways to stimulate the growth of new blood vessels, enhance tissue repair, and improve nerve function in the penis. These approaches hold the potential to provide longer-lasting and more natural solutions for ED.

COMBINATION THERAPIES

Researchers are also exploring the benefits of combining different treatment modalities. This includes combining PDE5 inhibitors like Cialis with other medications or therapies to enhance their effects. By targeting multiple aspects of the underlying causes of ED, combination therapies could offer a more comprehensive solution.

TELEMEDICINE AND REMOTE MONITORING

Advancements in telemedicine and remote monitoring are changing how patients access ED treatment. Telehealth platforms allow individuals to consult with healthcare providers remotely, reducing barriers to seeking help for sensitive issues like ED. This trend not only improves access to care but also enables more personalized and convenient treatment plans.

PSYCHOLOGICAL AND EMOTIONAL WELL-BEING

Recognizing the complex interplay between physical and psychological factors in ED, future treatments may focus more on addressing emotional well-being. Therapies that combine psychological counseling with medical interventions aim to provide holistic support for individuals struggling with both the physical and emotional aspects of ED.

CIALIS'S ROLE IN THE FUTURE

As research continues, Cialis remains a central player in the ED treatment landscape. Its unique extended duration of action and proven effectiveness position it as a versatile option for individuals seeking both as-needed and daily-use treatments. The insights gained from long-term use of Cialis can contribute to a deeper understanding of its impact on various aspects of sexual health and relationships.

NAVIGATING CONVERSATIONS AND SEEKING PROFESSIONAL ADVICE

Effective communication with partners and healthcare providers is essential when addressing erectile dysfunction and considering treatment options like Cialis. This chapter provides practical guidance on how to approach these conversations, seek professional advice, and make informed decisions for your sexual health.

TALKING TO YOUR PARTNER

1. **Choose the Right Time and Place:** Find a comfortable and private setting where

you and your partner can have an open and honest conversation about ED.

2. **Be Honest and Transparent:** Express your feelings and concerns openly. Explain how ED has affected you emotionally and physically, and emphasize that seeking treatment is a step toward improving intimacy and the relationship.

3. **Educate Your Partner:** Share information about ED and potential treatment options, including Cialis. Educating your partner can help them understand the condition and the steps you're taking to address it.

CONSULTING A HEALTHCARE PROVIDER

1. **Choose a Trusted Provider:** Seek out a healthcare professional you feel comfortable with. It could be a primary care physician, urologist, or a specialist in sexual health.

2. **Prepare for the Appointment:** Before the appointment, jot down your symptoms, concerns, and questions. This will ensure you cover all the relevant aspects during your visit.

3. **Discuss Your Medical History:** Provide your healthcare provider with a comprehensive medical history, including any medications you're taking and any underlying health conditions you have. This information is crucial for

making safe and effective treatment recommendations.

4. **Be Open About Lifestyle Factors:** Lifestyle choices, such as smoking, alcohol consumption, and stress levels, can contribute to ED. Be honest about these factors so your healthcare provider can offer tailored advice.

EXPLORING TREATMENT OPTIONS

1. **Consider Individual Needs:** Your healthcare provider will consider your overall health, medical history, and personal preferences when recommending treatment options.

2. **Discuss Cialis:** If appropriate, inquire about Cialis as a potential treatment. Ask about dosage options, administration

methods, and any potential interactions with other medications.

3. **Understand Risks and Benefits:** Your healthcare provider will explain the potential risks and benefits of the recommended treatment, including side effects and possible interactions.

EMPOWERING YOURSELF WITH KNOWLEDGE

1. **Stay Informed:** Take the time to research and understand your treatment options, including their mechanisms of action, potential side effects, and success rates.

2. **Seek Second Opinions:** If you're uncertain about the recommended treatment, don't hesitate to seek a

second opinion from another healthcare professional.

In conclusion, open and honest communication with both your partner and healthcare provider is essential for addressing erectile dysfunction effectively. By taking proactive steps to understand your condition and treatment options, you're empowering yourself to make informed decisions that positively impact your sexual health and overall well-being.

With this final chapter, we conclude our journey through the world of Cialis and its role in addressing the challenges of erectile dysfunction. Remember, seeking professional advice and tailored solutions is a crucial step toward regaining confidence, intimacy, and a fulfilling sexual relationship.

THE END

Made in the USA
Las Vegas, NV
27 December 2023

83546301R00020